Weight Burning

Your Calorie Burning Machine

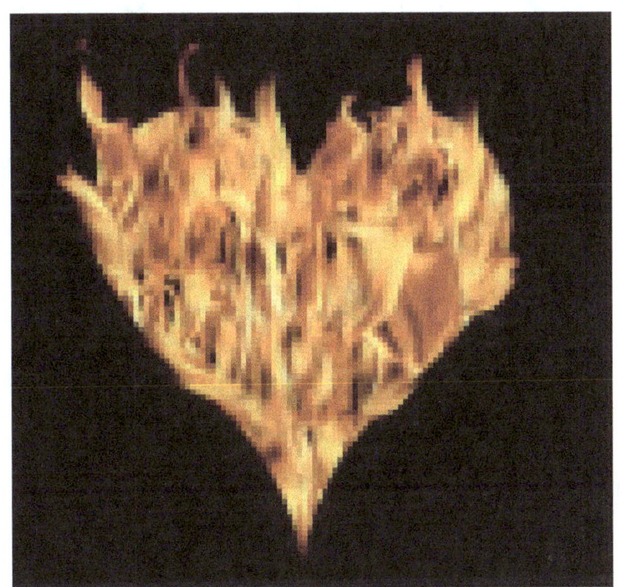

New Concepts

New Metabolism Booster Plan

New Innovative Exercise Plan

A twist on low-calorie plans is perfect for anyone with a SHORT-TERM WEIGHT LOSS GOAL or facing those LAST STUBBORN POUNDS.

Devoe Pelcher

Calorie Burner Your Way And Fast

Calorie A-La Carte Menu Plan

The New Metabolism Booster Plan

With A New Innovative Exercise Plan

"Turning Your Calorie Burning Machine to Maximum"

A new concept:

- ➢ **Individualizes Calorie Intake**
- ➢ **Increases Metabolism**
- ➢ **Burns Calories**
- ➢ **Promotes Fat Burning**

Bonus:

- ❖ **Anti-Aging Secrets**
- ❖ **Super Antioxidants**
- ❖ **Sample Menus**
- ❖ **Work Sheets**
- ❖ **Beneficial Spices**
- ❖ **Body Measurement Chart**
- ❖ **High Impact Exercise Plan**

A twist on low-calorie plans is perfect for anyone with a SHORT-TERM WEIGHT LOSS GOAL or facing those LAST STUBBORN POUNDS.

Table of Content

Weight Burner

Burn Calories Your Way

Devoe M. Pelcher

Copyrighted

12/24/2023

New and Innovative Plan

To

Boost your Metabolism

900-1800 *Calories A-La Carte Menu Plan*

Introduction:

The overall concept of this plan is to provide and allow an individual to go through their day as normal as possible, except how much and how often they consume food. This plan has been tested and yields an average of 3 lbs. of weight loss per week. In this plan, you are still allowed to eat what you want; only the quantity and amount will be the significant factor you must consider. To add quality to this plan, you should have fruit such as organic apples and grapefruits daily as snacks. In this plan, snacks play an important role. Snacks help to increase the amount of time you eat in a day; therefore, your metabolism is tricked into thinking it needs to burn calories. Doing this will cause the body to release abnormal fat reserves to burn as fuel. The body, in essence, never senses a need to store calories because it sees no need to store up for later. Therefore, you are always in a calorie-burning state.

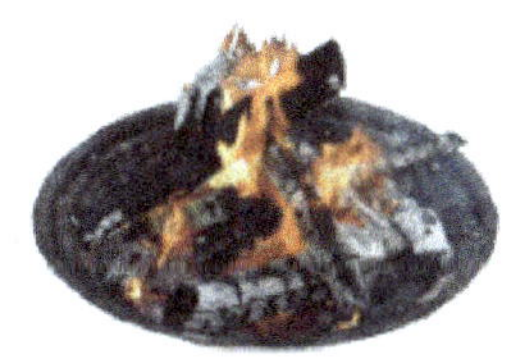

This plan will allow you to eat various foods or stick with a limited number of choices. No matter how you proceed, you are guided with a sliding calorie scale depending on how many calories you are to consume for that day. In this plan, you are given one free day a week to rest from the plan if you choose to take it, try to keep it to a minimum, and maintain control when you eat throughout the day. You are also given the opportunity to grade and track your mental state with five questions a day. To evaluate your accomplishment rate, answer each of five questions weighing 20 % for a perfect score of 100% for the day. The week is assessed similarly by averaging each day's accomplishment rate for an overall weekly accomplishment rate. There is also a chart to note your food intake and calorie count if you like to track your daily intake. Also, feel free to make daily notes on how things are going throughout the day and how you did for that day. There is also a list of 100 calories or less snacks provided.

Enjoy the plan, lose the weight, and enjoy the moment!

900-1800 Calories A-La Carte Menu Plan

First, you must remember to exercise and eat at least 5 to six times a day. If you begin to eat often, you will start to lose weight almost immediately. Now, I am not saying to eat more in quantity but to start eating more of the foods you should eat, like fruits, nuts, and vegetables, when you eat those 5 or 6 times a day. Science tells us that when you go on a diet or begin to starve yourself and eat significantly less food, your metabolism begins to slow down, and your body begins to store for survival.

Metabolism is the rate or speed at which your body burns food to carry out your body's necessary function. If you have a slow metabolism, your body burns food or calories very slowly; the opposite is true for a person with a fast metabolism. When consuming calories, a person with a slow metabolism will burn calories very slowly. The calories will not be turned into fuel but stored as fat because the calories are not used for bodily function. When the fat-burning machine begins to slow down, it is virtually impossible to lose weight. So what has to happen like a camp fire you must continue to put kindling on the fire to raise that fire to a roaring level.

For example, if you had a wood-burning furnace or even a campfire and you let the fire get down to the point where there were only ambers.

The ambers would not be enough to burn the amount of wood that you stack in the fire.

On the other hand, if the fire was blazing and you threw any amount of wood in it, there would be an immediate burning of the wood. That is the same with our bodies; if we have our metabolism turned up to a maximum level, we begin to immediately burn calories as they enter the body.

Non-fat, fresh, whole, unprocessed, and un-chemically altered food is the best fuel for the burning machine. These foods metabolize quickly and are as close to their natural form as possible. Your body is initially designed for these types of food. These foods remind me how easily paper will burn in a fire compared to a log.

When we talk about exercise, more is not always better. Building up to 45 min. to one hr. five times a week, slow and easy, is a great way to start an exercise program.

Today is your first day to start, not tomorrow or next week, but today. Dr. Peeke says there is no better day to greet the rest of your life than today.

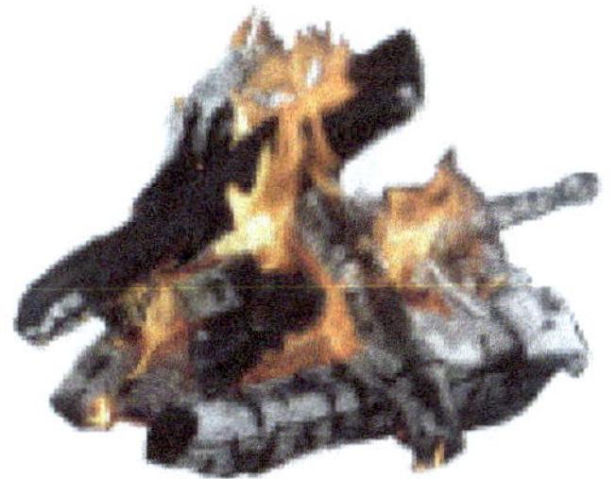

Discover my secret for getting out of the fat-burning plateau and back into the results zone.

A-La Carte Menu Plan

Things to consider when starting an exercise program would be:

Pick clothes that you will feel good wearing.

Schedule your workout so that last-minute interruptions will not sidetrack you.

Picking equipment that you will be working with may include but is not limited to some of the following:

Dumbbells

Weight Bench

Exercise Mat

Stability Ball

Resistance Tubing

Full Length Mirror

A Sturdy Chair

Play music that you like, that will keep you going and moving.

A-La Carte Menu Plan

If you have ever been on a diet before, you will love the A-La-Carte Menu Plan because you won't starve yourself, nor will you have to deprive yourself of the food that you like. Just remember moderation in all meals.

900-1800 Calories A-La Carte Menu Plan

Calories	900	1200	1500	1800
Breakfast choices	200-225	275-300	350-400	400-450
Early morning snacks	50-75	50	60-75	75-100
Lunch choices	350	375-425	450	500-600
Mid day snacks	50-75	50	75-100	90-125
Dinner choices	250-300	300-350	380-400	400-450
Late night snack	50	50	50-75	50-75

A-La Carte Menu Plan

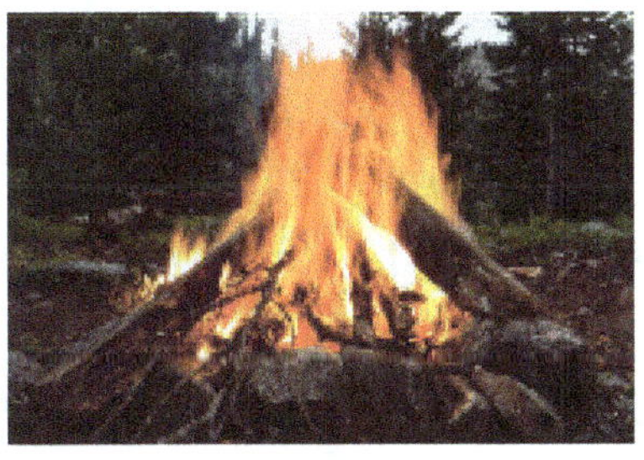

Calories in chart represent maximum numbers of calories for each meal for selected calorie plan.

A-La Carte Menu Plan

Sample Breakfast choices

Breakfast 1	Breakfast 2	Breakfast 3	Breakfast 4	Breakfast 5	Breakfast 6 Create your own
1 egg any way avg.90 cal	Two Fruits Any Kind	Hot or Cold Cereal	1-slice bacon 55 cal.	2-Pancakes w/jelly 170 cal.	
1 slice of bread of choice 90-110 cal.	2 glasses of water	2 glasses of water	1 slice toast 70 cal.	Two 8 oz. glasses of water	
1 glass of water			1 glass milk 100 cal.		
Avg. 290 cal.	Avg. 100 cal.		Avg. 120-200 cal.	Avg. 170 cal.	

Sample Snacks or research your own

Popcorn 2 cups 66,   Soup 1/2 cup 85,   1/2Can Fruit 50,
Grapefruit 30,   Peach 37,   Animal Crackers 5ea. 75,
Sugarless gum 10,   1 Apple 30, V8 8oz. 35, Yogurt Bar 97,
Cantaloupe 1 cup 58, 1 boiled egg, 5 saltine crackers,
1 pkg. cheese snack cracker, Slice toast & water, Cherry
tomatoes, 4 ea. ¼ tomato 30, 4 Grapefruit quarters 30,
3 oz. Celery stalks 30, 2 Rice cake 25, 1 or 2 Pickles

A-La Carte Menu Plan

Small Salads Sample

(Small Salad may substitute Lunch or Dinner)

Lettuce 30, tomato 30, carrots 34, red wine vinegar 0 =94

Lettuce 30, cucumber 25, tomato 30, 1 tbsp. salad dressing 80= 165

Large Salad Sample

(Large Salads: should only substitute Dinner)

Lettuce 30, tomato 30, carrots 34, cucumber 25, w/1oz of Turkey Ham or Luncheon Meat sliced and squared 36: Total=155 and w/dressing with 80 cal. =235

Lunch and Dinner:

(Maybe substituted with a small salad if desired)

Vegetables		Meats	
Squash	1 cup 40	Baked Pork Chop 3 oz. 200	
Spinach	1 cup 55	Veal	3 oz. 150
Can Soup	1 cup 150	Turkey	4-6 oz. 300
Frozen mixed Veg. 1 cup 100		Chicken Breast	4 oz. 180
Peas	1 cup 140	Frankfurter chicken 1ea. 75	

A-La Carte Menu Plan

Notes:

Spring water anytime   cal.=0

Fat free crackers anytime 5ea =50 calories.

 No Rye or whole grain.

Sugar cubes may be used: 8 calories each

Snack between meals.

All spices except salt allowed and encouraged.

Late night snacks could be crackers, popcorn or juice.

When eating fruit for breakfast, eat fruit only.

Juice added one time to any one meal during the day.

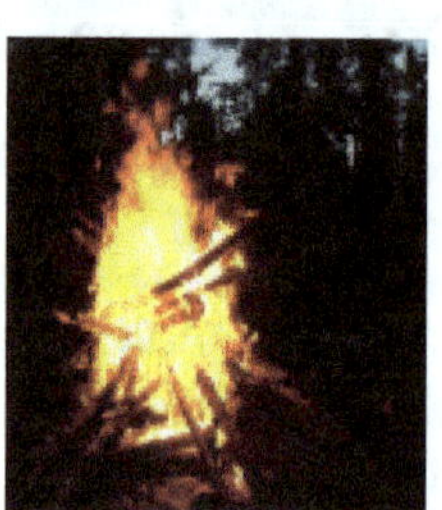

By no means possible, the information provided here is intended to be considered medical advice and promises no results when followed. Numbers provided may vary depending on sizes, quantities, and portions consumed.

A-La Carte Menu Plan

The Key to the Plan

2 days at 1200 calories, followed by 1 day at 1800 calories, then 2 days at 1500 calories, and the last day at 1800 calories ///

For even a Faster Metabolism, change to 3 days @ 1200 / 2 days @ 1800 calories / 2 days @ 1500 calories ///

Created by: Devoe Pelcher

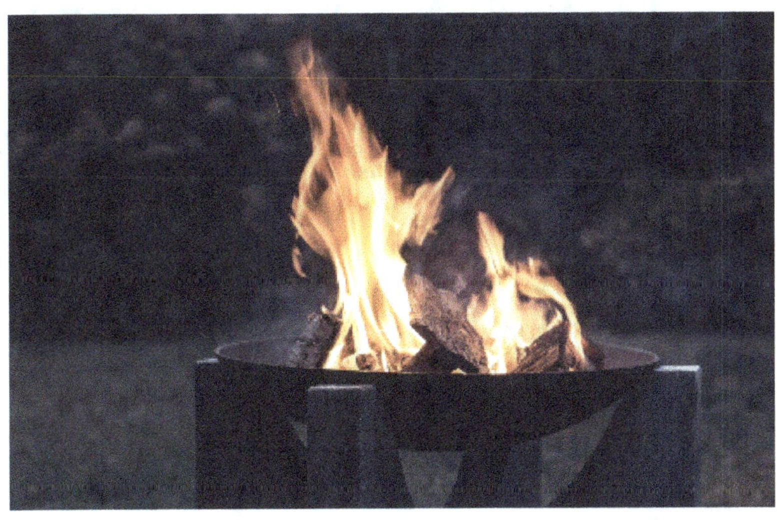

A-La Carte Menu Plan

This site has helpful eating habits for heart-healthy eating to help prevent cardiovascular disease

http://www.mayoclinic.com/health/heart-healthy-diet/NU00196

Your Own Calorie Burning Machine

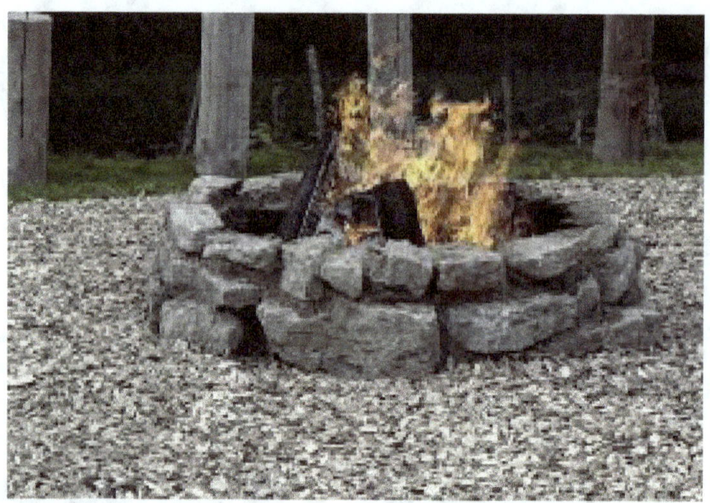

Determination: The act of deciding definitely and firmly, also a firm or fixed intention to achieve a desired end.

Beneficial Hints and Helpful Facts for Life Enhancement

a. To add detoxification to the plan, squeeze ½ lemon and two tablespoons of grade B maple syrup in 1 cup of water and drink in the morning after waking up.
b. Try to avoid graze during the day and eat distinct meals and snacks.
c. To ensure you get your snacks in, have your snacks ready on hand and in site.
d. Fruit is a perfect choice for a snack. Papaya, grapes, pineapple, and tomatoes will give you a wide range of needed enzymes.
e. It doesn't matter what time you wake up in the morning; that is your breakfast.
f. Exercise every day that you are on the plan. Incorporate exercises that work problem areas.
g. Shelled seafood has weight loss qualities.
h. Don't let other liquids replace your water intake.
i. Take fruit and vegetable pills to supplement your requirement needs, if necessary.
j. Get an adequate amount of sleep. If you sit at work all day, you can get away with decreased sleep; if you are very active all day, you need to increase your sleep to give you more time for rebuilding.

k. For people with a poor appetite, I suggest you individualize the plan according to your tolerance and tastes. Also, B vitamins help to increase the appetite.

l. There are 100-calorie snacks available now in supermarkets.

m. When buying baggies for lunch, also consider purchasing the snack baggies.

n. Protein and Carbohydrates differ in that protein originates from live animals with eggs and eyes, such as fish, meat, chicken, etc., and carbohydrates originate from plants. Examples are grains, beans, breads, sugars, potatoes, avocadoes, etc.

o. For proper food, combining protein, an acid base, and starch, an alkaline base, should be kept separate. Either can be combined with vegetables and either can be combined with legumes/beans.

p. Generally, you will find that most fried foods are protein and fat, and most baked foods are carbohydrates and fats.

q. Building muscle keeps your metabolism revived, so you burn more calories while at rest.

r. Most of the people who utilize the plan found out that it takes about 2-3 weeks to turn the metabolism-burning machine on maximum, and after the plan, like myself, found out that just because you are not on the plan, you will still be losing weight for about 2-3 weeks.

s. Most people found out that after getting on the plan, the plan became a habit to them rather than a chore in life, and they began to make better food choices that resulted in better overall health.

900-1800 Calories A-La Carte Menu Plan

16 Weeks Accomplishment Rate Sheets

Calorie Goal _______   Week #   Day Initial   Percent

Overall evaluation of Week #   _______   _______   _______%

	YES	NO	Comment
Stayed within calorie limit	____	____	____________________
Completed all meals	____	____	____________________
Completed all snacks	____	____	____________________
Exercised	____	____	____________________
Consumed $\geq$32 oz. of water	____	____	____________________

Calorie Goal _______   Week #   Day Initial   Percent

Overall evaluation of Week #   _______   _______   _______%

	YES	NO	Comment
Stayed within calorie limit	____	____	____________________
Completed all meals	____	____	____________________
Completed all snacks	____	____	____________________
Exercised	____	____	____________________
Consumed $\geq$32 oz. of water	____	____	____________________

900-1800 *Calories A-La Carte Menu Plan*

Accomplishment Rate Sheet

Calorie Goal _______ 　　　　Week #　　Day Initial　　Percent

Overall evaluation of Week #　_______　________　________%

　　　　　　　　　　　　　YES　　NO　　　　Comment

Stayed within calorie limit　____　____　________________

Completed all meals　　　　____　____　________________

Completed all snacks　　　　____　____　________________

Exercised　　　　　　　　____　____　________________

Consumed $\geq$32 oz. of water____　____　________________

Calorie Goal _______ 　　　　Week #　　Day Initial　　Percent

Overall evaluation of Week #　_______　________　________%

　　　　　　　　　　　　　YES　　NO　　　　Comment

Stayed within calorie limit　____　____　________________

Completed all meals　　　　____　____　________________

Completed all snacks　　　　____　____　________________

Exercised　　　　　　　　____　____　________________

Consumed $\geq$32 oz. of water____　____　________________

900-1800 Calories A-La Carte Menu Plan

Accomplishment Rate Sheet

Calorie Goal _______   Week #   Day Initial   Percent

Overall evaluation of Week #   _______   ________   ________%

	YES	NO	Comment
Stayed within calorie limit	____	____	_________________
Completed all meals	____	____	_________________
Completed all snacks	____	____	_________________
Exercised	____	____	_________________
Consumed $\geq$32 oz. of water	____	____	_________________

Calorie Goal _______   Week #   Day Initial   Percent

Overall evaluation of Week #   _______   ________   ________%

	YES	NO	Comment
Stayed within calorie limit	____	____	_________________
Completed all meals	____	____	_________________
Completed all snacks	____	____	_________________
Exercised	____	____	_________________
Consumed $\geq$32 oz. of water	____	____	_________________

900-1800 Calories A-La Carte Menu Plan

Accomplishment Rate Sheet

Calorie Goal _______   Week #   Day Initial   Percent

Overall evaluation of Week #   _______   ________   ________%

	YES	NO	Comment
Stayed within calorie limit	____	____	________________
Completed all meals	____	____	________________
Completed all snacks	____	____	________________
Exercised	____	____	________________
Consumed $\geq$32 oz. of water	____	____	________________

Calorie Goal _______   Week #   Day Initial   Percent

Overall evaluation of Week #   _______   ________   ________%

	YES	NO	Comment
Stayed within calorie limit	____	____	________________
Completed all meals	____	____	________________
Completed all snacks	____	____	________________
Exercised	____	____	________________
Consumed $\geq$32 oz. of water	____	____	________________

900-1800 Calories A-La Carte Menu Plan

Accomplishment Rate Sheet

Calorie Goal _______   Week #   Day Initial   Percent

Overall evaluation of Week #   _______   _______   _______%

	YES	NO	Comment
Stayed within calorie limit	____	____	_________________
Completed all meals	____	____	_________________
Completed all snacks	____	____	_________________
Exercised	____	____	_________________
Consumed $\geq$32 oz. of water	____	____	_________________

Calorie Goal _______   Week #   Day Initial   Percent

Overall evaluation of Week #   _______   _______   _______%

	YES	NO	Comment
Stayed within calorie limit	____	____	_________________
Completed all meals	____	____	_________________
Completed all snacks	____	____	_________________
Exercised	____	____	_________________
Consumed $\geq$32 oz. of water	____	____	_________________

900-1800 Calories A-La Carte Menu Plan

Accomplishment Rate Sheet

Calorie Goal _______   Week #   Day Initial   Percent

Overall evaluation of Week #   _______   _________   ________%

	YES	NO	Comment
Stayed within calorie limit	____	____	_________________
Completed all meals	____	____	_________________
Completed all snacks	____	____	_________________
Exercised	____	____	_________________
Consumed $\geq$32 oz. of water	____	____	_________________

Calorie Goal _______   Week #   Day Initial   Percent

Overall evaluation of Week #   _______   _________   ________%

	YES	NO	Comment
Stayed within calorie limit	____	____	_________________
Completed all meals	____	____	_________________
Completed all snacks	____	____	_________________
Exercised	____	____	_________________
Consumed $\geq$32 oz. of water	____	____	_________________

900-1800 Calories A-La Carte Menu Plan

Accomplishment Rate Sheet

Calorie Goal _______   Week #   Day Initial   Percent

Overall evaluation of Week #   _______   _________   ________%

	YES	NO	Comment
Stayed within calorie limit	____	____	__________________
Completed all meals	____	____	__________________
Completed all snacks	____	____	__________________
Exercised	____	____	__________________
Consumed $\geq$32 oz. of water	____	____	__________________

Calorie Goal _______   Week #   Day Initial   Percent

Overall evaluation of Week #   _______   _________   ________%

	YES	NO	Comment
Stayed within calorie limit	____	____	__________________
Completed all meals	____	____	__________________
Completed all snacks	____	____	__________________
Exercised	____	____	__________________
Consumed $\geq$32 oz. of water	____	____	__________________

900-1800 *Calories A-La Carte Menu Plan*

Accomplishment Rate Sheet

Calorie Goal _______   Week #   Day Initial   Percent

Overall evaluation of Week #   _______   _______   _______%

                     YES   NO   Comment

Stayed within calorie limit ____   ____   ___________________

Completed all meals   ____   ____   ___________________

Completed all snacks   ____   ____   ___________________

Exercised   ____   ____   ___________________

Consumed $\geq$32 oz. of water____   ____   ___________________

Calorie Goal _______   Week #   Day Initial   Percent

Overall evaluation of Week #   _______   _______   _______%

                     YES   NO   Comment

Stayed within calorie limit ____   ____   ___________________

Completed all meals   ____   ____   ___________________

Completed all snacks   ____   ____   ___________________

Exercised   ____   ____   ___________________

Consumed $\geq$32 oz. of water____   ____   ___________________

A-La Carte Menu Plan

Additional 100 calorie and below

Snack to choose from

1. Twenty chocolate-covered raisins. 87 cal.

2. Half a slice of angel food cake with 1 tablespoon thawed, frozen light whipped topping and one maraschino cherry. 94 cal.

3. Five Starburst Fruit Chews. 100 cal.

4. One whole graham cracker, broken into two squares. Top one square with 1/4 oz-piece milk chocolate and one large marshmallow. Top with the other square and microwave for about 12 seconds. 90 cal.

5. Two 1-inch squares chocolate fudge. 86 cal.

6. Fruit mix: three dried apricot halves, four almonds and one tablespoon chocolate chips. 100 cal.

7. One frozen waffle toasted and topped with two sliced strawberries and 1 tablespoon whipped cream. 99 cal.

8. 1/2 cup Cocoa Puffs cereal with 1/4-cup skim milk. 81 cal.

9. Three gingersnaps. 80 cal.

10. 6-oz tub Yoplait White Chocolate Strawberry nonfat yogurt. 100 cal.

11. Half a banana, with 1 tablespoon each chocolate syrup and thawed, frozen light whipped topping. 99 cal.

12. Two fun-size Nestle Butterfinger bars. 68 cal.

13. 1 cup sugar-free hot chocolate with 2 tablespoons miniature marshmallows. 66 cal.

14. Two caramel corn cakes. 90 cal.

15. 3/4-oz serving baked potato chips (7 to 12 chips) with 2 tablespoons fat-free onion dip. 85 cal.

16. Four wheat crackers with 1-oz reduced-fat cheddar cheese. 87 cal.

17. Half a baked potato, with 1 tablespoon each reduced-fat sour cream and salsa. 98 cal.

18. Six medium pretzel twists with 2 tablespoons mustard. 91 cal.

19. Seven medium shrimp with lemon to taste. 70 cal.

20. Half a medium onion bagel. 97 cal.

21. Three toasted 1/4-in.-thick slices Italian bread, topped with 3 tablespoons chopped tomatoes, 1/2 teaspoon olive oil, minced garlic and fresh basil. 79 cal.

22. Four pieces plain Melba toast. 78 cal.

23. Twenty-Five pistachio nuts. 85 cal.

24. Half a baked flour tortilla with 1 oz avocado and 1 tablespoon salsa. 88 cal.

25. 6 cups light microwaveable popcorn. Season to taste. 93 cal.

26. Half a toasted whole-wheat English muffin with one teaspoon reduced-fat chunky peanut butter. 85 cal.

27. Three dill pickles. 36 cal.

28. One baked hash-brown potato patty, with 1 tablespoon ketchup. 79 cal.

29. 2 tablespoons humus on a quarter toasted pita. 93 cal.

30. Half a baked sweet potato mashed with 1 teaspoon each honey and diet margarine. 96 cal.

31. Skinny cafe latte (2 oz brewed espresso with 1 cup steamed skim milk). 91 cal.

32. 1/2 cup cooked couscous and 2 teaspoons grated Parmesan cheese. 100 cal.

33. 1 cup serving canned condensed tomato soup, prepared with water. 85 cal.

34. 1-oz light roasted turkey breast, with 1 teaspoon yellow mustard and one leaf romaine lettuce on one slice toasted light whole-wheat bread. 94 cal.

35. Two low fat chocolate chip cookies (store-bought) heated in microwave for 10 seconds. 90 cal.

36. 1/2 cup prepared plain instant oatmeal, with 2 tablespoons frozen blueberries and cinnamon to taste. 82 cal.

37. One slice toasted raisin bread with 1 tablespoon fat-free cream cheese. 86 cal.

38. 1/4-cup egg substitute omelet, filled with 1 tablespoon reduced-fat cheddar cheese and 1/4 cup diced tomatoes. 88 cal.

39. 1 cup green tea with 2 teaspoon sugar. 30 cal.

40. Ten baby carrots with 2 tablespoons fat-free ranch dressing. 90 cal.

41. 1/2 cup each green and red bell pepper sliced and dipped in 2 tablespoons light Thousand Island dressing. 80 cal.

42. 1/2 cup canned pineapple chunks, packed in juice. 75 cal.

43. One chocolate-dipped strawberry. 62 cal.

44. Five small celery ribs stuffed with 2 teaspoons peanut butter and 1 tablespoon raisins. 100 cal.

45. Half a medium grapefruit with 1 teaspoon sugar. 38 cal.

46. One each sliced medium tomato and red onion with 2 tablespoons low-fat Italian salad dressing. 100 cal.

47. 1/2-cup low-fat cottage cheese blended with 4 tablespoons fresh blueberries. 100 cal.

48. One small baked apple with 1 1/2 tablespoons light pancake syrup. 97 cal.

49. 1/2 cup light vanilla ice cream with 2 tablespoons frozen raspberries. 100 cal.

50. 1/4 cup cooked soybeans (edamame) seasoned to taste. 64 cal

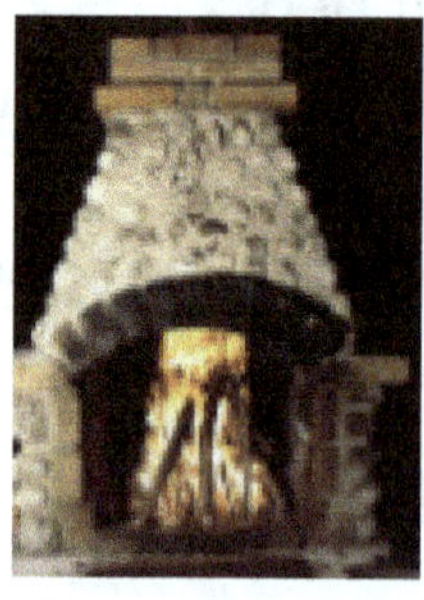

Consistency : Firmness of constitution of character to continue and endure in a repetitive manner, marked by harmony, regularity, or steady continuity : free from variation or contradiction.

A-La Carte Menu Plan

100 Calories, 75 Calories, 50 Calories, 25 Calories Suggestions

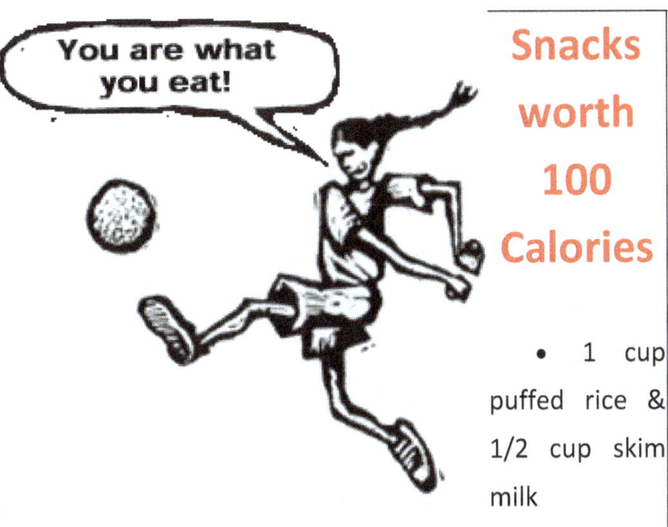

- 1 cup puffed rice & 1/2 cup skim milk
- 1 cup puffed wheat & 1/2 cup skim milk
- 1/2 English muffin & 1/2 tsp butter
- 1 slice toast & 1 tsp jelly
- 1 rice cake & 1 T. peanut butter
- 1/2 cup vanilla yogurt
- 1/2 cup low-fat cottage cheese
- 1 cup skim milk
- 1 large apple
- 1 pear
- 1 small banana
- 1 cup chicken rice soup
- 1 cup beef barley soup
- 1 oz. mozzarella cheese

- 1 cup minestrone soup
- 1 cup turkey vegetable soup
- 1 cup chicken noodle soup
- 1 cup peas & carrots
- 1/2 cup prune juice
- 4 oz. shrimp
- 2 oz turkey
- 1/2 cup sherbet
- 1 cup apple juice
- 10 walnut halves
- 15 almonds
- 4 brazil nuts
- 30 pistachios
- 1/2 cup oatmeal
- 1 cup fruit cocktail
- 1 ear corn
- 1 tea matzo
- 1 tortilla
- 1 small pita (1 oz.)
- 1 small oatmeal cookie
- 1 tsp. peanut butter
- 1 frozen fruit bar
- 1/2 cup fat-free frozen yogurt

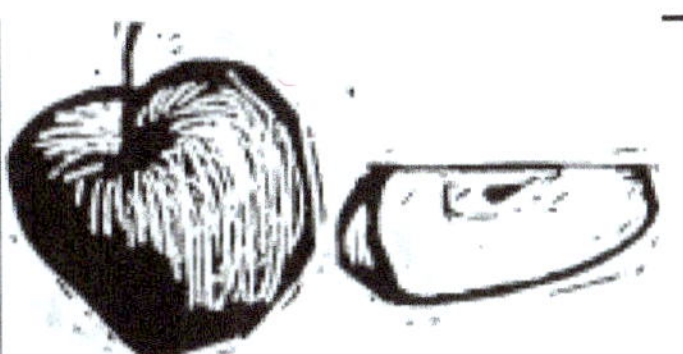

75 Calorie Munchies

- 1 slice bread
- 3 cups air-popped popcorn
- 1 slice American cheese (3/4 oz.)
- 4 raw kumquats
- 1 Milano cookie
- 2 shortbread cookies
- 1 medium apple
- 1 large pineapple slice
- 1 hardboiled egg

25 Calorie Tidbits

- 5 stalks celery
- 5 zucchini sticks
- 1 cup raw green beans
- 1 large carrot
- 1 tomato
- 1 small plum
- 1 prune
- 1 apricot
- 1 stalk broccoli
- 1/2 cup beets
- 9 brussel sprouts
- 1 cup shredded cabbage
- 1/2 cup spinach (cooked)
- 1 large green pepper
- 12 radishes
- 2 whole cucumbers
- 1 cup cauliflower
- 7 oz. lettuce
- 2 large dill pickles
- 2 large olives
- 1 saltine
- 1 marshmallow

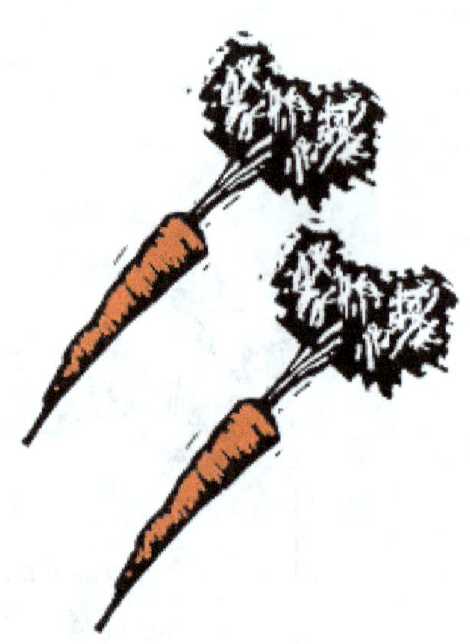

A-La Carte Menu Plan

More 100 calorie and below

Snack to choose from

1 oz. 40 % bran flakes, 90 calories.

1 oz. cream cheese, 100 calories
1 raw apple, 80 calories

1 12 oz. diet soda, 0 calories
3 raw apricots, 50 calories

1 fried egg, 90 calories
1 cooked artichoke, 55 calories

6 slices of cucumber, 5 calories
1 cup asparagus, 50 calories

1 omelet, 100 calories
1 homemade biscuit, 100 calories

1 oz. feta cheese, 75 calories
1 small or medium banana, 100 calories

1 hard-boiled egg, 75 calories
1 cup cooked bean sprouts, 25 calories

1 fish stick from frozen, 70 calories
1 cup canned beef broth, 15 calories

6 oz. brewed coffee, 0 calories
1 cup cooked collards raw, 25 calories

3 oz. raw clams, 65 calories

1 cup cooked beets, 55 calories

3 oz. canned clams, 85 calories
1 cup raw blackberries, 75 calories

1 tsp. cinnamon, 5 calories
12 fluid oz. club soda, 0 calories

1 tsp. chili powder, 10 calories
1 cup raw blueberries, 80 calories

1 cup Canned clam chowder, 80 calories
1 cup cooked broccoli, 50 calories

1 cup chicken rice soup, 60 calories
2 slices of light chicken roll, 90 calories

1 1.6 oz. roasted chicken drumstick, 75 calories
1 cup of brown gravy, 80 calories

1 cup cooked steamed eggplant, 25 calories
1 cup buttermilk, 100 calories

1 brownie with nuts and icing, 100 calories
1 ounce of blue cheese, 100 calories

1 cup cooked Brussels sprouts, 65 calories
1 pat of salted butter, 35 calories

1 slice cracked-wheat bread, 65 calories

1 cup cooked cabbage, 30 calories
1 cup raw cabbage, 15 calories

½ of a raw cantaloupe, 95 calories

1 cup cooked collards from frozen, 60 calories
3 cooked chicken livers, 90 calories

1 cup cooked carrots, 70 calories
20 sweet raw cherries, 100 calories

1 cup raw carrots, 30 calories
1 cup sour red raw canned cherries, 90

1 tbsp catsup, 15 calories
20 plain cheese crackers, 100 calories

1 cup cooked cauliflower, 35 calories
1 cup raw celery, 20 calories

10 frozen grapes, 100 calories

2 cheese crackers with peanut butter, 80 calories
1 ear white or yellow corn from frozen, 60 calories
1 cup chicken gravy from dry mix, 85 calories
1 cup canned chicken noodle soup, 75 calories
2 brown and serve sausage links, 100 calories
1 pkt. mix and eat cream of wheat, 100 calories
1 pkt. of instant cooked corn grits, 80 calories

1 cup canned beef noodle soup, 85 calories
1 tbsp. blue cheese salad dressing, 75 calories
1 cubic inch of cheddar cheese, 70 calories

1 cup canned chicken chow mein, 95 calories

Endeavor : To attempt (as the fulfillment of an obligation) by exertion of effort to complete a task with a set purpose. <endeavors to finish the race>

900-1800 *Calories A-La Carte Menu Plan*

A-La Carte Menu Plan

My Personal Daily Log for Three Weeks on The Plan.

This log of events is intended to show that everyone makes mistakes and that you can overcome them with a few mental changes and adjustments. This log will show you that you can also turn your metabolism burner on despite making a few mistakes. So don't be so hard on yourself that you give up before seeing the results. I can tell you that I am still burning calories, and I have a calorie-burning machine on my hands. So, in reality, you can turn your burning machine to the max and get the results that you are looking for. It will not be and is not intended to be a fast weight loss method.

What is not present here is the exercise routine that you should incorporate into the plan. I might revise this book to include my exercise routine during the plan. There should be an exercise routine because you want to maintain your muscles during this time. One way not to lose your muscle mass is to exercise. You may also see the muscle's weight, but there will also be definition and less fat present. That is a good thing!

Persistent : Existing for a long or longer than usual time or continuously: as a : retained beyond the usual period <a persistent leaf> b : continuing without change in function or structure and continuing to exist despite interference or treatment <a persistent cough>

A-La Carte Menu Plan

My log follows:

Started Weight at 198 lbs.

Week 1 Goals:

A. **Maintain the Daily Limits**
B. **Exercise everyday**
C. **3 lbs. weight loss**

WK1-Monday   Goal 1200 calories

06:55 hrs. cereal with milk and a banana   110 + 45

1130 , snacked on a boiled egg and 1 slice of raisin toast 90 + 100

1330 hrs. serving of pinto beans, serving of spinach and a corn bread muffin   230

2030 1 fillet of catfish and water   165

Overall evaluation of Monday: 80%

	YES	NO	Comment
Stayed within calorie limits	X		740 cal. Out of 1200
Completed all meals	X		
Completed all snacks		X	
Exercised	X		
Consumed $\geq$32 oz. of water	X		

A-La Carte Menu Plan

WK1-Tuesday   Goal 1200 calories

0800 Peanut butter and jelly sandwich with water

                              70+70+40+50

1100   24 cheese nips   *100*

1400 3 oz meat loaf / ¼ cup rice, ¼ muffin 200+50+40

1600 Catfish fillet and rice   *160 + 50*

1800 1 Chicken breast   *180*

2200 10 Grapes   *100*

Overall evaluation of Tuesday: 100%

	YES	NO	Comment
Stayed within calorie limits	X		1115 cal. Out of 1200
Completed all meals	X		
Completed all snacks	X		
Exercised	X		
Consumed ≥32 oz. of water	X		

A-La Carte Menu Plan

WK1-Wednesday   Goal 1800 calories

0630   Raisin Bran cereal with milk and sugar   300

1120 Kernel corn and small portion of meat loaf 175 + 75

1300 Short Salad (lettuce, slice tomatoes, cheese, dressing)

200 + cheese 114 + 170/ Mountain Dew

1639 3 cups popcorn   100

2130 2 oz. Pasta   212

3 shrimps   321

2330 Peanut butter and Jam sandwich

Wednesday evaluation:

I started early this morning, hungry upon waking up. I might have been awakened by hunger and decided to eat Raisin Bran cereal since this was 1800 calorie day. I was hungry at about 0930 but waited because I had no snacks close by me while I was at my workstation. I decided to have a lunch salad with a soda instead of water.

Snack time came fast, and I did not know what to snack on. I decided to pop popcorn and eat 3 cups. I mentally felt like I needed to exercise or something. So, I walked to fulfill that urge while exerting that extra energy. I got Busy during the evening and ate dinner at 2130.

I performed misc. tasks at home, had a late-night snack at about 2330, and went to bed a little after midnight.

A-La Carte Menu Plan

Overall evaluation of Wednesday: 80%

	YES	NO	Comment
Stayed within calorie limits		X	1876 cal. Out of 1800
Completed all meals	X		
Completed all snacks	X		
Exercised	X		
Consumed ≥32 oz. of water	X		

WK1-Thursday Goal 1500 calories

0930 2 slices raisin toast	200
2 over light eggs	180
2 slices of bacon	110
8 oz. water	
1145 1 apple	30
1415 6 oz ground beef steak	
w/mushroom and gravy and	
¼ cup brown rice	480 + 25 + 50
16 oz pineapple juice	260
2130 Mixed fruit cup	100

A-La Carte Menu Plan

Thursday evaluation:

I woke up around 0600, exercised, and reorganized the store room. I did not get a chance to eat until 0930, but I was able to drink liquids. I had a late-morning snack that consisted of an apple. Everything has shifted in time because of the late breakfast. Lunch was at 1415, and my portions and quantity of items were too much, creating a high-calorie intake for lunch. That left me only a few choices for the rest of the day. I am up to 1345 cal. The solution to this issue is implementing a trade-off system by exercising and burning off some of those extra calories collected.

I walked around the building at a very brisk pace for 5 minutes. You can burn approximately five calories per minute, equating to 25 calories. It is not much, but If done four times, it will equate to 100 calories gone, diminished, not there and walked about 50 calories off. 1335-50=1285 so far for the day. Looking back over today, I see that my breakfast did not need to be that large. The cafeteria had a sale this morning for $1.99, which I could not pass up. The solution was to split the breakfast so that some of it would be for an early morning snack. I went out and purchased snacks that were prepackaged for a total of 100 calories. Later, I got busy until 2130, took a break, and ate a mixed fruit bowl without eating anything for dinner.

A-La Carte Menu Plan

Overall evaluation of Thursday: 80%

	YES	NO	Comment
Stayed within calorie limits	X		1435 cal. Out of 1500
Completed all meals		X	
Completed all snacks	X		
Exercised	X		
Consumed $\geq$32 oz. of water	X		

0030 Catfish snack   *100*

WK1-Friday   Goal   1500 calories

0630 Bowl Oatmeal w/margarine and sugar   *240*

0945 Reese's Snacksters   *100*

1215 Broiled Cod fish, 90   rice, 50 steamed vegetables 75

    ¼ roll   20

1730 slice of watermelon   *75*

2030 ½ Fillet catfish   *75*

    Broccoli and cheese   *100*

Friday evaluation:

I had an early morning snack before going to bed. I woke up at 0530, which was pretty early for me. However, I exercised and started my day. I ate at about 0630. I weighed myself and lost 3 lbs., which was good for four days. I found myself looking for something to fulfill the calorie limits for the day. I had a late snack before dinner and no snack before or after dinner.

Overall evaluation of Friday: 100%

	YES	NO	Comment
Stayed within calorie limit	X		1435 cal. Out of 1500
Completed all meals	X		
Completed all snacks	X		
Exercised	X		
Consumed >32 oz. of water	X		

Overall evaluation of week 1: 88% accomplishment rate

I incorporated food from fast food restaurants, home cooking, and cafeterias this week. Weight lost as of Friday was 3lbs. Fish was the primary meat not by choice but because of availability. I felt no extreme hunger. I did not get hunger alerts, which I saw I needed to pay attention to to stay true to the plan. Saturday and Sunday were free days for me. I realized that neither day should have been free. I had yet to establish enough discipline to go two days without a regiment. I had a domino party Saturday, ate a lot of food, and drank plenty of liquids, not water, but sodas.

A-La Carte Menu Plan

Evaluation of week 1continue:

Sunday, I ate leftovers which I felt was just a carryover from Saturday. Two days performed at 100%, three days at 80%., two days ate without control. Manage to lose the 3lbs. goal weight by day 5. I accomplished an overall consistency rate of 88% in staying true to the plan.

Week 2

Reminder

900-1800 Calories A-La Carte Menu Plan

Calories	900	1200	1500	1800
Breakfast choices	200-225	275-300	350-400	400-450
Early morning snacks	50-75	50	60-75	75-100
Lunch choices	350	375-425	450	500-600
Mid day snacks	50-75	50	75-100	90-125
Dinner choices	250-300	300-350	380-400	400-450
Late night snack	50	50	50-75	50-75

A-La Carte Menu Plan

Calories in chart represent maximum numbers of calories for each meal for selected calorie plan.

Week 2

Goals:

A. Exercise with weights
B. Drink water w/ lemon juice every morning for detoxification.
C. Start a vitamin regiment.
D. 3 lbs. weight lost.

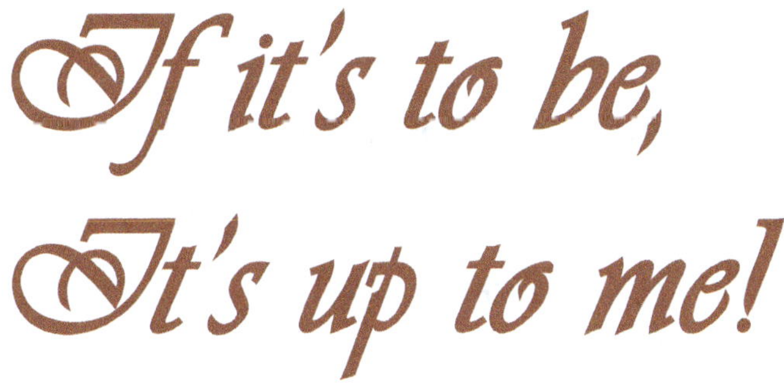

WK2-Monday   Goal: 1200 calories

0400 Early morning snack, Bowl of Oatmeal   100

0800 Bowl Oatmeal   100

1045 Hershey's snacksters   100

1212 1 Chicken Wing   250

1600 5 swiss cookies   50

1800 2 Hot chicken wings w/ rice   600

Monday evaluation :

I started my day by waking up early at around 4:00 AM and had oatmeal as my early morning snack. I felt hungry throughout the day but only consumed the calories prescribed in my diet plan. I attribute my hunger to overeating during the weekend.

Overall evaluation of Monday: 80%

	YES	NO	Comment
Stayed within calorie limit	X		1150 cal. Out of 1200
Completed all meals	X		
Completed all snacks		X	
Exercised	X		
Consumed $\geq$32 oz. of water			

WK2-Tuesday   Goal: 1200 calories

0800 beef pattie	*200*
1030 snackers	*100*
1230 Soup	*200*
corn fritters	*225*
1630 snackers	*100*
1900 Noodles	*250*
2230 Four chocolate chips	*400*

Overall evaluation of Tuesday: 80%

Tuesday evaluation: Failed to chart breakfast and late night snack.

	YES	NO	Comment
Stayed within calorie limit		X	1475 cal. 275 over1200
Completed all meals	X		
Completed all snacks	X		
Exercised	X		
Consumed $\geq$32 oz. of water	X		

WK2-Wednesday   Goal: 1800 calories

0800 30 grapes	*300*
1030 snackers	*100*
1200 Oatmeal	*100*
1600 Goldfish w/peanut-jelly	*100*
1545 3 cups of popcorn	*100*
2100 2 Sodas	*320*
2300 1 hot dog	*80*

Overall evaluation of Wednesday: 100%

Wednesday evaluation: Followed the plan well today. Encountered no problems

	YES	NO	Comment
Stayed within calorie limit	X		1100 cal. Out of 1800
Completed all meals	X		
Completed all snacks	X		
Exercised	X		
Consumed $\geq$32 oz. of water	X		

WK2-Thursday   Goal: 1500 calories

0830	Early snack	100
	8 oz. pineapple-orange juice	100
0930	omelet	350
1100	1 cup of pinto beans w/BBQ sauce	100
1545	red beans and rice	180
	corn muffin	130
1715	Four cookies	80

Thursday evaluation: Decided to have an early morning snack and late breakfast to try to get in a snack at least 1 hr.

Overall evaluation of Thursday: 100%

	YES	NO	Comment
Stayed within calorie limit	X		1190 cal. Out of 1200
Completed all meals	X		
Completed all snacks	X		
Exercised	X		
Consumed $\geq$32 oz. of water	X		

WK2-Friday   Goal   1500 calories

0730 watermelon   *100*

0815 4 oz. cup water w/ ½ lemon

1100 pear   *100*

1245 6 oz .slice Roast beef   *380*

1700 keebler 100 cal snack   *100*

2000 ½ baked potato w/tomatoes and cheese   350

Friday   evaluation: I started off with fruit this morning to make it easier for the digestive system. Also, incorporating water with lemon juice starts the detoxification stage that you can implement in the plan. I did not exercise this morning. Weight this morning was 190lbs. I met goal of 3 lbs. for the week. My total weight now is 190lbs.

Overall evaluation of Friday: 100%

	YES	NO	Comment
Stayed within calorie limit	X		1030 cal. Out of 1500
Completed all meals	X		
Completed all snacks	X		
Exercised	X		
Consumed ≥32 oz. of water	X		

Overall evaluation of week 2: Manage to lose the 3lbs goal weight by Week 2 day 5. I started drinking lemon water late in the week. Began to take vitamins and did not start the weight training. I accomplished an overall consistency rate of 92% in staying true to the plan.

A-La Carte Menu Plan

Week 3

Goals:

A. Exercise with weights
B. Drink water w/ lemon juice every morning for detoxification.
C. Continue the vitamin regiment.
D. Weight less than 190
E.

WK3-Monday   Goal 1200 calories

0700 ½ lemon squeezed into ½ cup of water

0900 ½ omelet w/ham, cheese, sausage and pepper   350

1000 Peach Green Tea   70

1130 lemon bar   unknown approx. 350

1415 Mushroom, zucchini and onions   200

1515 1/8 lbs of chicken thigh   150

1745 100 cal snack   100

2100 3 J/B Tacos   495

A-La Carte Menu Plan

Monday evaluation: Meals were too large. There were too many snacks and too close together. This would have been a good day for an 1800 cal. Day.

Overall evaluation of Monday: 40%

	YES	NO	Comment
Stayed within calorie limit		X	1730 cal. 550 > 1200
Completed all meals	X		
Completed all snacks		X	
Exercised		X	
Consumed >32 oz. of water	X		

Your Calorie Burning Machine

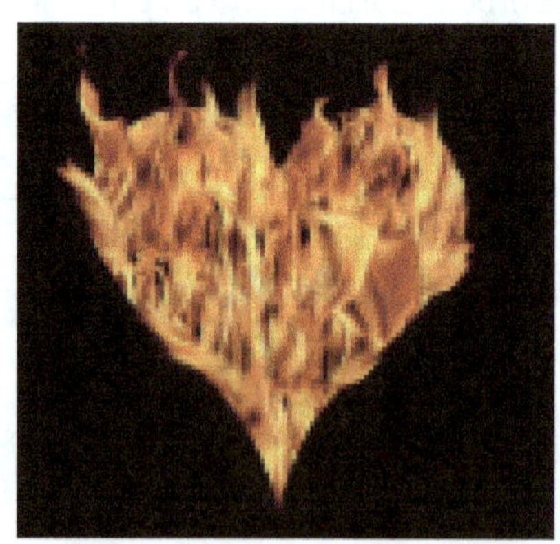

WK3-Tuesday   Goal 1200 calories

0800 ½ lemon squeezed into ½ cup of water

0830 Peanut butter sandwich   *200*

1230 2 boiled eggs   *140*

    Snacker Reeses   *100*

1530 Snacker Hershey's   *100*

1930 3 Taquilas chicken & beef   *500*

2100 Juice   *140*

Overall evaluation of Tuesday: 100%

	YES	NO	Comment
Stayed within caloric limit	X		1180 cal. Out of 1200
Completed all meals	X		
Completed all snacks	X		
Exercised	X		
Consumed $\geq$32 oz. of water	X		

WK3-Wednesday   Goal 1800 calories

0800 ½ lemon squeezed into ½ cup of water

0830 Peanut butter and jam sandwich	250
1230 1 cup lentils	250
1400 100 calorie snacker	100
1900 1 fillet cat fish	250
2200 1 hamburger pattie	238

Overall evaluation of Wednesday: 80%

	YES	NO	Comment
Stayed within calorie limit	X		1800 cal. Out of 1200
Completed all meals	X		
Completed all snacks	X		
Exercised		X	
Consumed ≥32 oz. of water	X		

WK3-Thursday

Goal 1800 calories substituted for 1200 day that I went over

0800 Oatmeal   *100*

1230 1 slice cake   *250*

1500 Red Beans and Rice   *180*

10 oz Pepsi   *100*

1700 100 calorie snack   *100*

1845 1 chicken leg   *230*

½ cup green beans   *70*

½ cup mashed potatoes   *120*

Overall evaluation of Thursday: 80%

	YES	NO	Comment
Stayed within calorie limit	X		1150 cal. Out of 1800
Completed all meals	X		
Completed all snacks	X		
Exercised	X		
Consumed ≥32 oz. of water	X		

WK 3 Friday   Goal   1200 calories

0800 Bowl of Corn Flakes	100
1030 3 p and j on double crackers	100
1300 Mushroom soup	240
2 ground beef meat pies	500
1700 100 calorie snack	100
1900 1 chicken Breast	180

Overall evaluation of Friday: 80%

	YES	NO	Comment
Stayed within calorie limit		X	1120 cal. 12 > 1200
Completed all meals	X		
Completed all snacks	X		
Exercised	X		
Consumed ≥32 oz. of water	X		

Overall evaluation of week 3:

On the first day, I started by exceeding Monday's calorie limit by 550 calories.

I will compensate by substituting an 1800 day for 1200 and see the results. I seemed to have had some trouble remembering to snack. A possible solution to remembering to snack is having the snack before me waiting on the snack time. One of the 1800 days was not met; I fell short of about 650 calories, which was okay because of the 1200-calorie day that I went over by 550.

Your Calorie Burning Machine

Week 4: I am not counting calories to the extent of the past three weeks. I do unintentionally notice the quantity of food that I will consume during one setting and try to make sure that I continue to get my snacks in for the day. My future plan is to maintain a less than 2000 calorie per day plan. My basal caloric rate to maintain the weight lost is 1900 calories. If I have dinner late I will eliminate the late snack.

Week 5&6: Continued as week 4, realized that I have met my goal and is time now to really concentrate on not losing any more weight and to create an exercise routine and incorporate weights into the plan in order to bulk up. Continue detoxification with the lemon routine. My program will then be finished.

Enjoy the plan, lose the weight, and enjoy the moment!

A-La Carte Calorie Menu Plan

Sample Day Menu

Breakfast

1 slice

Toast with Peanut Butter, Jelly and Fruit Juice [Calories 275]

1slice,
1slice whole wheat bread
2 tsp peanut butter
2 tsp low-calorie jelly
1/2 cup fruit juice

Toast the bread and top with peanut butter and jelly. Serve with fruit juice.

Snack Suggestion

1 serving fruit [Calories 70]

Lunch

Subway Sandwich & Yogurt [Calories 250]
Subway: 6" Deli Turkey Breast Sandwich
1 small low-fat yogurt

1 oz ham wrapped round and a handful of carrot sticks
[Calories 40]

Dinner

Quick Chicken Wrap & Salad [Calories 297]
1 soft flour tortilla (6-8" dia)
2 oz shredded cooked chicken
1/2 oz low-fat shredded cheese
1 sliced tomato, 1/2 tsp dried herbs
1 cup salad leaves
1 tbsp fat-free or low-fat dressing

Layer tortilla with sliced tomato and chicken and top with the cheese. Sprinkle herbs over and roll up. Heat in a toaster oven for 3 minutes or microwave for 60 seconds.

Snack Suggestion

4 oz fruit cup in juice [Calories 55]

Extra Allowance

1 Cup fat-free milk (or equivalent)

Total Calories   **Daily Calories: 1082**

Sample Breakfast Menus

Breakfast Menus

1 egg any way   avg.90

1 slice raisin bread   90

Grapefruit Juice   <u>100</u>

                280

Fruit

1- grapefruit   88

1 banana   124

1 Apple   <u>80</u>

                192

Hot or cold Cereal   120

Milk   100

1 slice of Toast   70

1slice bacon   <u>55</u>

                325

Substitute breakfast items: * 2 Boiled Eggs 45 calories each

.   * Instant Grits 1 oz. 100

                * 2 Plain Pancakes w/ jelly 170

Commitment: An agreement or pledge to do something in the future

Your Calorie Burning Machine

Opinions about Calorie *Burner* Plan

Note: To preserve privacy, all identifying names have been removed.

I really liked the booster diet to start. It not only helps get a few pounds off right away, it also gives you a great sense of how much food you should be eating daily. Even now, when I am in a slump or plateau, I will switch back to the booster even if only for 1 week and my weight starts moving again.

This is my 1st completed week on the low calorie plan and exercise every other day. It was hard at first, but starting to get the hang of it. I just weighed myself and I have lost 4lbs! I have been stalled at 155 pounds for 8 weeks, so getting over this weight plateau has really "boosted" my confidence!!

I'm doing the Happy Dance!!!!
Been on the Low Calorie Booster Plan for one week since joining here. I am so HAPPY to say I am down 5 pounds for the week and, wait for it, I'm not hungry!!!.

Down another 5 pounds this week. That's 11 pounds in 2 weeks.....Wow! didn't realize the Booster diet would give me such a boost hehehe....

I weighed in this morning at 167 pounds, which really surprised me as that is a loss of 4 pounds this week. I didn't really feel like I was depriving myself and didn't expect to lose anything like that. This is one happy girl!!!!!

```
Wow! I've just weighed myself and I can't believe
it. I've lost 6 pounds. I've never lost 6 pounds
in my life before. I checked 3 times and it's
true. This booster diet is awesome!!!
```

Enduring : To remain firm under suffering or misfortune without yielding <though it is difficult, we must endure>, to undergo (as a hardship) especially without giving in, to continue in the same state

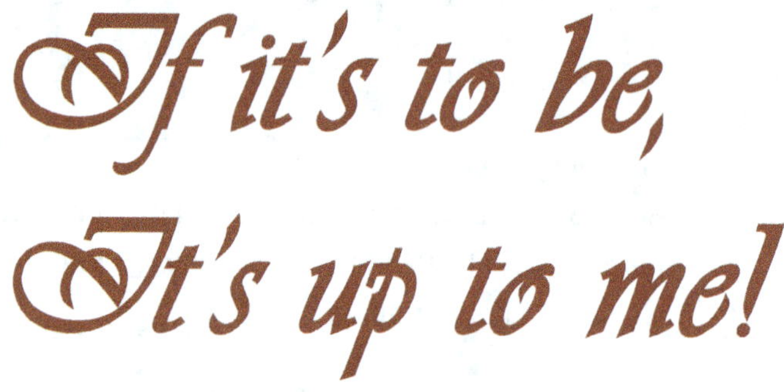

Commitment: An agreement or pledge to do something in the future

A-La Carte Calorie Menu Plan

Calorie Work Sheet

(Breakfast/Snack/Lunch/Snack/Dinner/ opt. Snack)

Week # _____ Day # _____   Week # _____ Day # _____

Time   Food   Calories   Time   Food   Calories

Calorie Work Sheet
(Breakfast/Snack/Lunch/Snack/Dinner/ opt. Snack)

Week # _____ Day # _____   Week # _____ Day # _____

Time	Food	Calories	Time	Food	Calories
_____	_____________	_____	_____	_____________	_____
_____	_____________	_____	_____	_____________	_____
_____	_____________	_____	_____	_____________	_____
_____	_____________	_____	_____	_____________	_____
_____	_____________	_____	_____	_____________	_____
_____	_____________	_____	_____	_____________	_____
_____	_____________	_____	_____	_____________	_____
_____	_____________	_____	_____	_____________	_____
_____	_____________	_____	_____	_____________	_____
_____	_____________	_____	_____	_____________	_____
_____	_____________	_____	_____	_____________	_____

Note:

Calorie Work Sheet
(Breakfast/Snack/Lunch/Snack/Dinner/ opt. Snack)

Week # _____ Day # _____   Week # _____ Day # _____

Time	Food	Calories	Time	Food	Calories
____	__________	____	____	__________	____
____	__________	____	____	__________	____
____	__________	____	____	__________	____
____	__________	____	____	__________	____
____	__________	____	____	__________	____
____	__________	____	____	__________	____
____	__________	____	____	__________	____
____	__________	____	____	__________	____
____	__________	____	____	__________	____
____	__________	____	____	__________	____
____	__________	____	____	__________	____

Note:

Calorie Work Sheet
(Breakfast/Snack/Lunch/Snack/Dinner/ opt. Snack)

Week # _____ Day # _____   Week # _____ Day # _____

Time   Food   Calories   Time   Food   Calories

____   ___________   ____   ____   ___________   ____

____   ___________   ____   ____   ___________   ____

____   ___________   ____   ____   ___________   ____

____   ___________   ____   ____   ___________   ____

____   ___________   ____   ____   ___________   ____

____   ___________   ____   ____   ___________   ____

____   ___________   ____   ____   ___________   ____

____   ___________   ____   ____   ___________   ____

____   ___________   ____   ____   ___________   ____

____   ___________   ____   ____   ___________   ____

____   ___________   ____   ____   ___________   ____

____   ___________   ____   ____   ___________   ____

Note:

Calorie Work Sheet

(Breakfast/Snack/Lunch/Snack/Dinner/ opt. Snack)

Week # _____ Day # _____   Week # _____ Day # _____

Time	Food	Calories	Time	Food	Calories
____	__________	_____	____	__________	_____
____	__________	_____	____	__________	_____
____	__________	_____	____	__________	_____
____	__________	_____	____	__________	_____
____	__________	_____	____	__________	_____
____	__________	_____	____	__________	_____
____	__________	_____	____	__________	_____
____	__________	_____	____	__________	_____
____	__________	_____	____	__________	_____
____	__________	_____	____	__________	_____
____	__________	_____	____	__________	_____
____	__________	_____	____	__________	_____

Note:

Calorie Work Sheet
(Breakfast/Snack/Lunch/Snack/Dinner/ opt. Snack)

Week # _____ Day # _____   Week # _____ Day # _____

Time	Food	Calories	Time	Food	Calories
_____	_____________	_____	_____	_____________	_____
_____	_____________	_____	_____	_____________	_____
_____	_____________	_____	_____	_____________	_____
_____	_____________	_____	_____	_____________	_____
_____	_____________	_____	_____	_____________	_____
_____	_____________	_____	_____	_____________	_____
_____	_____________	_____	_____	_____________	_____
_____	_____________	_____	_____	_____________	_____
_____	_____________	_____	_____	_____________	_____
_____	_____________	_____	_____	_____________	_____
_____	_____________	_____	_____	_____________	_____

Note:

Calorie Work Sheet

(Breakfast/Snack/Lunch/Snack/Dinner/ opt. Snack)

Week # _____ Day # _____   Week # _____ Day # _____

Time	Food	Calories	Time	Food	Calories

Note:

Calorie Work Sheet
(Breakfast/Snack/Lunch/Snack/Dinner/ opt. Snack)

Week # _____ Day # _____   Week # _____ Day # _____

Time	Food	Calories	Time	Food	Calories

Note:

Calorie Work Sheet

(Breakfast/Snack/Lunch/Snack/Dinner/ opt. Snack)

Week # _____ Day # _____   Week # _____ Day # _____

Time	Food	Calories	Time	Food	Calories
_____	____________	_____	_____	____________	_____
_____	____________	_____	_____	____________	_____
_____	____________	_____	_____	____________	_____
_____	____________	_____	_____	____________	_____
_____	____________	_____	_____	____________	_____
_____	____________	_____	_____	____________	_____
_____	____________	_____	_____	____________	_____
_____	____________	_____	_____	____________	_____
_____	____________	_____	_____	____________	_____
_____	____________	_____	_____	____________	_____
_____	____________	_____	_____	____________	_____
_____	____________	_____	_____	____________	_____

Note:

Calorie Work Sheet

(Breakfast/Snack/Lunch/Snack/Dinner/ opt. Snack)

Week # _____ Day # _____   Week # _____ Day # _____

Time	Food	Calories	Time	Food	Calories

Note:

Calorie Work Sheet

(Breakfast/Snack/Lunch/Snack/Dinner/ opt. Snack)

Week # _____ Day # _____   Week # _____ Day # _____

Time	Food	Calories	Time	Food	Calories

Note:

If it's to be,
It's up to me!

Accomplishment and Calorie Rate Sheet Combine

Week #   Day   % Calorie Goal

Overall evaluation_____ ________ _____ _________

	YES	NO	Comment
Stayed within calorie limit	____	____	____________
Completed all meals	____	____	____________
Completed all snacks	____	____	____________
Exercised	____	____	____________
Consumed $\geq$32 oz. of water	____	____	____________

Calorie Work Sheet

(Breakfast/Snack/Lunch/Snack/Dinner/ opt. Snack)

Week # _____ Day # _____   Week # _____ Day # _____

Time	Food	Calories	Time	Food	Calories
____	__________	____	____	__________	____
____	__________	____	____	__________	____
____	__________	____	____	__________	____
____	__________	____	____	__________	____
____	__________	____	____	__________	____

                      Week #   Day   % Calorie Goal

Overall evaluation____ _______ ____ _________

                         YES   NO   Comment

Stayed within calorie limit   ____   ____ _____________

Completed all meals   ____   ____ _____________

Completed all snacks   ____   ____ _____________

Exercised   ____   ____ _____________

Consumed $\geq$32 oz. of water ____   ____ _____________

Calorie Work Sheet
(Breakfast/Snack/Lunch/Snack/Dinner/ opt. Snack)

Week # ____ Day # ____   Week # ____ Day # ____

Time	Food	Calories	Time	Food	Calories
____	__________	____	____	__________	____
____	__________	____	____	__________	____
____	__________	____	____	__________	____
____	__________	____	____	__________	____
____	__________	____	____	__________	____
____	__________	____	____	__________	____

Accomplishment and Calorie Rate Sheet Combine

Week #   Day   % Calorie Goal

Overall evaluation_____ ________ _____ _________

	YES	NO	Comment
Stayed within calorie limit	____	____	___________
Completed all meals	____	____	___________
Completed all snacks	____	____	___________
Exercised	____	____	___________
Consumed $\geq$32 oz. of water	____	____	___________

Calorie Work Sheet

(Breakfast/Snack/Lunch/Snack/Dinner/ opt. Snack)

Week # _____ Day # _____   Week # _____ Day # _____

Time	Food	Calories	Time	Food	Calories
____	__________	____	____	__________	____
____	__________	____	____	__________	____
____	__________	____	____	__________	____
____	__________	____	____	__________	____
____	__________	____	____	__________	____

Accomplishment and Calorie Rate Sheet Combine

                    Week #   Day   % Calorie Goal

Overall evaluation____ _______ ____ ________

	YES	NO	Comment
Stayed within calorie limit	____	____	________
Completed all meals	____	____	________
Completed all snacks	____	____	________
Exercised	____	____	________
Consumed $\geq$32 oz. of water	____	____	________

Calorie Work Sheet
(Breakfast/Snack/Lunch/Snack/Dinner/ opt. Snack)

Week # ____ Day # ____   Week # ____ Day # ____

Time	Food	Calories	Time	Food	Calories
___	______	____	___	______	____
___	______	____	___	______	____
___	______	____	___	______	____
___	______	____	___	______	____
___	______	____	___	______	____

Accomplishment and Calorie Rate Sheet Combine

Week #   Day   % Calorie Goal

Overall evaluation______ _________ ______ __________

	YES	NO	Comment
Stayed within calorie limit	____	____	____________
Completed all meals	____	____	____________
Completed all snacks	____	____	____________
Exercised	____	____	____________
Consumed >32 oz. of water	____	____	____________

Calorie Work Sheet

(Breakfast/Snack/Lunch/Snack/Dinner/ opt. Snack)

Week # _____ Day # _____   Week # _____ Day # _____

Time	Food	Calories	Time	Food	Calories
____	____________	____	____	____________	____
____	____________	____	____	____________	____
____	____________	____	____	____________	____
____	____________	____	____	____________	____
____	____________	____	____	____________	____

Accomplishment and Calorie Rate Sheet Combine

Week #   Day   % Calorie Goal

Overall evaluation______   ________ _____ _________

	YES	NO	Comment
Stayed within calorie limit	____	____	___________
Completed all meals	____	____	___________
Completed all snacks	____	____	___________
Exercised	____	____	___________
Consumed ≥32 oz. of water	____	____	___________

Calorie Work Sheet
(Breakfast/Snack/Lunch/Snack/Dinner/ opt. Snack)

Week # ____ Day # ____   Week # ____ Day # ____

Time	Food	Calories	Time	Food	Calories
____	________	____	____	________	____
____	________	____	____	________	____
____	________	____	____	________	____
____	________	____	____	________	____
____	________	____	____	________	____
____	________	____	____	________	____

Weight Burner Body Measurement Chart

The goal is to gain inches while losing pounds

Date: _________________________

Weight: _________________________

Circumference Measurements (See below for instructions):

Neck: _________________________

Biceps: _________________________

Wrist: _________________________

Chest: _________________________

Waist: _________________________

Hips: _________________________

Thigh: _________________________

Calf: _________________________

Burn fat and build muscle

How to Measure

Waist

Measure your waist without holding the tape too tightly (or too loosely). As a rough guide, your waist is the narrowest part of your trunk, or approximately 1 inch above your belly button.

Hips

Measure the hips around the fullest part of your buttocks with your heels together.

Thighs

Measure the upper thighs, just below where the buttocks merge into the back thigh.

Chest

Measure around the fullest part of chest

Nuggets about Cinnamon, Flaxseed and Nutmeg

Cinnamon

The sweet and spicy flavor of cinnamon has been used by many different cultures for its medicinal properties for hundreds, even thousands, of years.

One of the most talked about benefits of cinnamon relates to type 2 diabetes. A study published in the journal Diabetes Care found that half a teaspoon of cinnamon a day significantly reduces blood sugar levels in people with type 2 diabetes. It also reduces triglyceride, LDL cholesterol, and total cholesterol levels among this group.

Cinnamon's other benefits include:

- Supports digestive function
- Constricts and tones tissues
- Relieves congestion
- Relieves pain and stiffness of muscles and joints
- Relieves menstrual discomfort
- Blood-thinning compounds that stimulate circulation
- Anti-inflammatory compounds that may relieve arthritis
- Helps prevent urinary tract infections, tooth decay and gum disease
- It's a powerful anti-microbial agent that can kill E. coli and other bacteria

Nutmeg

Nutmeg is another spice that has a variety of healing properties and can be used in a wide range of dishes during the holidays and all year long. It is useful for:

- Insomnia (nutmeg can produce drowsiness so it should be taken when you have a chance to relax or sleep)
- Anxiety   Toothaches (nutmeg oil)
- Calming muscle spasms   Lowering cholesterol
- Nausea and vomiting   Increasing circulation
- Indigestion   Improving concentration
- Diarrhea   Lowering blood pressure
- Joint pain and gout
- Male infertility and impotence

Flaxseed and Flaxseed Oil

Flaxseed or the flaxseed oil which is extracted from the seed is rich in magnesium, omega-3 essential fatty acids, potassium, B vitamins, protein, zinc and fiber. The taste is pleasant and can be mixed with water or any vegetable or fruit juice. The seeds can be grinded in a coffee grinder and be added to soups, salads, yogurt baked goods and cereals. Studies show that it has reduced the pain associated with arthritis. It has also found to reduce blood cholesterol and triglyceride levels, Flaxseed has also helped reduced the hardening effects of cholesterol on cell membranes.

Beneficial Enzymes for Life Enhancement

Digestive enzymes and metabolic enzymes.

Digestive enzymes mainly fall into three categories which are amylase, protease, and lipase. These enzymes are secreted along the gastrointestinal tract and break down foods, enabling the nutrients to be absorbed into the bloodstream to be use in various bodily functions

Amylase, found in saliva and in the pancreatic and intestinal juices, break down specific types of sugars. For example, lactase breakdown milk sugar (lactose), maltase break down cane and beet sugar (sucrose).

Protease, found in the stomach juices and also in the pancreatic and intestinal juices, help to digest protein.

Lipase, found in the stomach and pancreatic juices, and also present in fats in foods, aid in fat digestion.

Metabolic enzymes are enzymes that the whole body uses that catalyze the various chemical reactions within the cells, such as energy production and detoxification. Each body tissue has it own specific set of metabolic enzymes, but two particularly important metabolis enzymes are superoxide dismutase (SOD) and catalase.

SOD (superoxide dismutase) is an antioxidant that protects the cells by attacking a common free radical, superoxide. Superoxide dismutase occurs naturally in a variety of food sources, including barley grass, broccoli, Brussels sprouts, cabbage, wheatgrass, and most green plants.

Catalase breaks down hydrogen peroxide, a metabolic waste product, and liberates oxygen for the body to use.

The late Dr. Edward Howell, a physician and pioneer in enzymes research, called enzymes the "sparks of life". They are essential for digesting food, for stimulating the brain, for providing cellular energy, and for repairing all organs, cells, and tissues. Each enzyme has a specific function in the body that no other enzyme can fulfill. The life we now know could not exist without the actions of enzymes. While the body manufactures a supply of enzymes, it can also obtain enzymes from food. Unfortunately, enzymes are extremely sensitive to heat. Even low to moderate heat (118 degrees Fahrenheit or above) destroys most enzymes in food, so to obtain enzymes from the diet, one must eat raw foods. Eating raw foods or, alternatively, taking enzyme supplements, help prevents depletion of the body's own enzymes and thus reduce the stress on the body. Enzymes can be found in many different foods, from both plant and animals sources. Avocados, papayas, pineapples, bananas, and mangos are all high in enzymes. Sprouts are the richest source.

Your Calorie Burning Machine

The overall concept of this plan is to provide and allow an individual to go through their day as normal as possible, except how much and how often they consume food. This plan utilizes your own calorie-burning furnace that you already have to burn calories. This plan shows you how to turn it on and off when you want to. This plan has been tested and yields an average of 3 lbs. of weight loss per week. In this plan, you are still allowed to eat what you want. So there will be no starving yourself; only the quantity and the amount will be the significant factor in this plan that you must consider. If you do feel starved, like I did on one of the days. I came to the conclusion as to why. You may find your reason as well.

Disclaimer

The information in this book is provided as an information resource only, and is not to be used or relied on for any diagnostic or treatment purposes. This information does not create any patient-physician relationship, and should not be used as a substitute for professional diagnosis and treatment. I expressly disclaims responsibility, and shall have no liability, for any damages, loss, injury, or liability whatsoever suffered as a result of your reliance on the information contain in this book. The information presented is not and should not be construed to be legal, medical or consulting advice. References and links to third parties do not constitute an endorsement or warranty of any kind. All research, trial, logs and opinions are not intended to replace medical advice and should review the information carefully with their professional health care provider. I will not be liable for any direct, indirect, consequential, special, exemplary or other damages arising from your use of this material presented. This information is not intended to provide medical information. Should you have a medical condition, promptly see your own medical doctor. This information is not a personalized medical diagnosis or patient advice. This disclaimer is to encourage you to make informed decisions about your health and inform you that this is for informational purposes only and should not be used in place of an actual professional visit or advice from a professional and that the information provided is to be used at your own risk.